ACCEPT THE CHAllENGE

Published by Gordon Visionary Publishing, LLC

ISBN: 978-1-967645-14-5
Library of Congress Control Number: 2025926980
Cover Design By: Dori Dubin
Edited by: Gordon Visionary Publishing, LLC

Printed in the United States of America
First Edition: December 2025
For permissions and inquiries, contact: gordonvisionarypublishing@gmail.com

Your Purchase Makes a Difference
We appreciate your support for Gordon Visionary Journals' mission! A portion of the proceeds of each journal sold goes to the Gordon Family Foundation and Trust, reflecting our commitment to service and education by investing in future leaders, one scholarship at a time.

This journal belongs to:

____

Make this YOURS!

About this Journal

The **Accept the Challenge** guided journal provides a 30-day plan to support the learning of and mastering of five techniques related to accepting any challenge you may encounter in life using a different approach or enhancing your current approach.

The guided journal includes thought-provoking writing prompts and exercises that will provide opportunities to change how you approach challenges, increase your positive thinking and decision-making skills, use of personal space and time, what opportunities to take advantage of, value of relationships, and to build more productive habits related to addressing life's challenges.

As you embark on the Accept the Challenge journey, remember you will have an opportunity to strengthen specific skill sets related to addressing challenges, learn an innovative approach to challenges, be empowered to integrate the techniques into your day-to-day activities, and have a planned method for tackling challenges.

Daily, you will:

- learn about five techniques necessary to accept the challenge
- practice applying the five accept the challenge techniques to different scenarios
- integrate the five techniques into your day-to-day routines
- reflect on and track your progress throughout the process
- strengthen your resiliency skills and mental well-being
- embrace challenges with a positive mindset

Now let's meet the Visionary Team that will help you on your Accept the Challenge Journey.

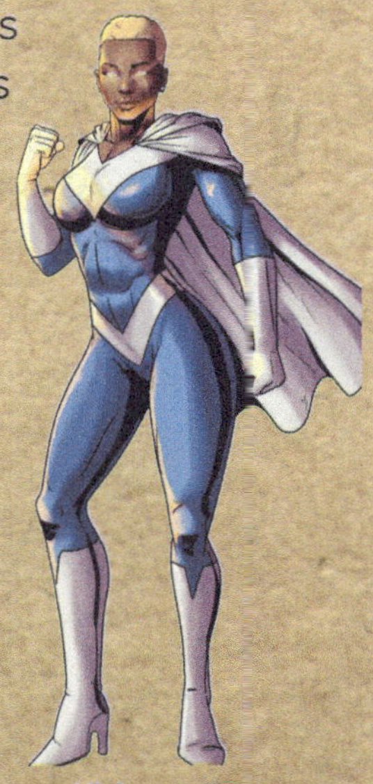

Visionary Team

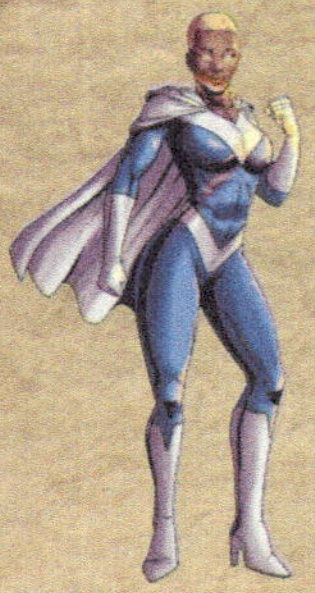

Visionary

I am **Visionary**. I embody optimism, forward-thinking, and boldness, guiding you to see the bigger picture. My role is to inspire, uplift, and encourage you, pushing you beyond your limits. **Picture where you could be in a year from now. Believe in the possibility and Embrace the Challenge!**

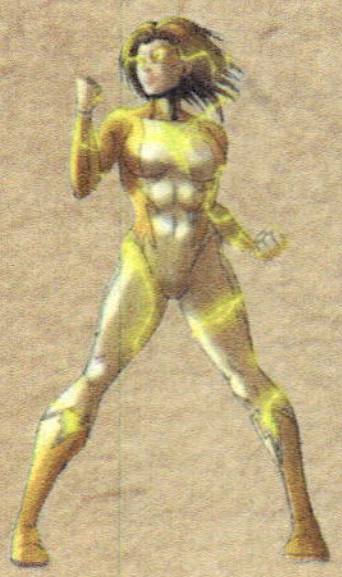

Energy

I am **Energizer**. I symbolize limitless enthusiasm, boundless energy, and a spark of passion. I inspire you, ignite your motivation, and offer affirmation. I'm here to invigorate you when you're feeling stuck. **Let's get moving! You already possess the inner energy needed to power through the Challenge.**

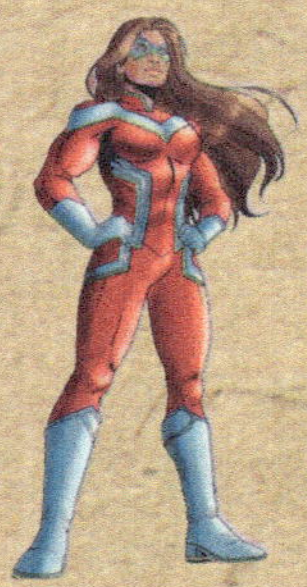

Challenger

I am **Challenger**. I embody boldness, assertiveness, and thought-provoking questions. I push you beyond your limits, encourage you to step out of your comfort zone, and tackle challenges directly with courage. **Picture being confrontational yet compassionate. Together, we will confront fears, failures, and even the fear of success. You are unstoppable, so embrace the Challenge.**

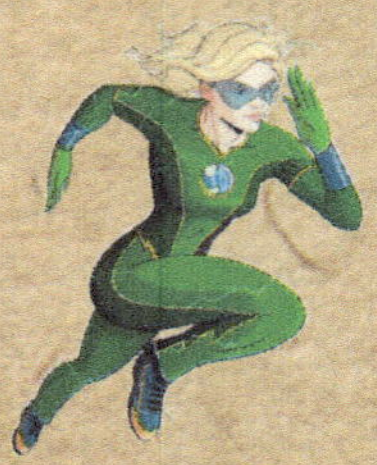

Activator

I am **Activator.** I embody the spirit of action and the drive to make things happen without lingering too long. I inspire you to embrace your boldness, decisiveness, and fearlessness. **Challenge yourself to seize opportunities and take a step each day toward achieving our goals.**

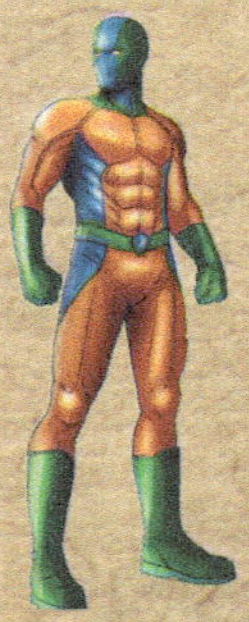

Excusor

I am **Excusor**. I embody the unwanted distractions and the voices that hinder your progress. I urge you to overcome obstacles, resist interruptions, and manage your time effectively. **Stay focused on your goals by saying no or postponing those things that do not propel you forward in facing the Challenge.**

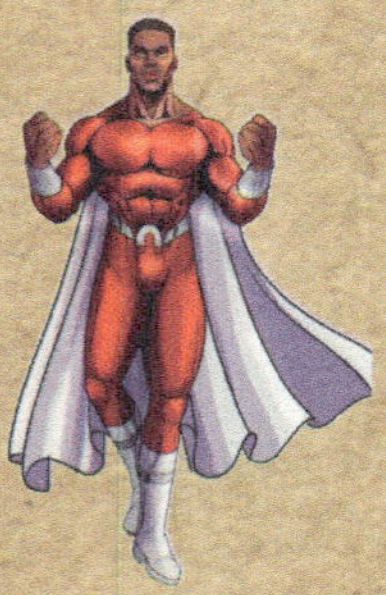

Gravitator

I am **Gravitator**. I embody focus, grounding force, and a source c alignment. I inspire you to remain caln to center yourself, and trust yoı intuition. Steer clear of chaos an concentrate on what genuinel matters and who matters. **Align you energy with your priorities and sta focused on the Challenge ahead.**

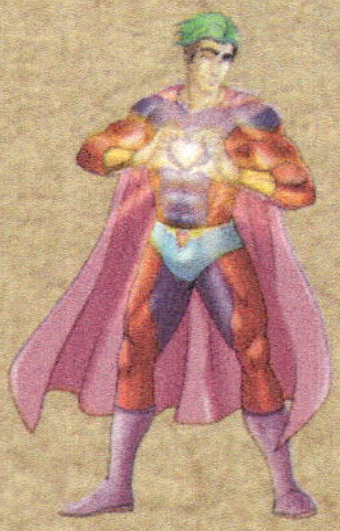

Grateful

I am **Grateful**. I represent gratitude and appreciation. I inspire you to pause, reflect, and give thanks. **Take a moment to be still, be reflective, be grateful daily through the Challenge.**

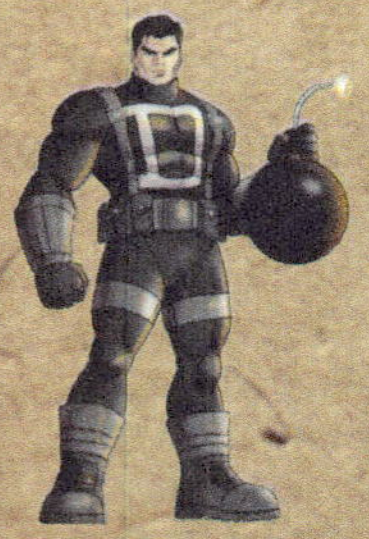

Detonator

I am **Detonator.** I embody motivatio daring actions, fearlessness, ar unwavering drive. I will encourage yo to shatter self-doubt and embrac risk-taking. **Don't let anything ho you back; let's dive in wholeheartedl Give this Challenge everything you'v got!**

ACCEPT THE CHALLENGE PLEDGE

Today, I welcome the challenge and I pledge to:

- Embrace the challenge
- Identify the desired change
- Let in anything/any person I need to change
- Excuse myself from anything/any person hinder my change
- Activate and engage in opportunities need to change
- Gravitate and engage with others that support the change
- Track and share my progress until I reach the desired change
- Repeat the process

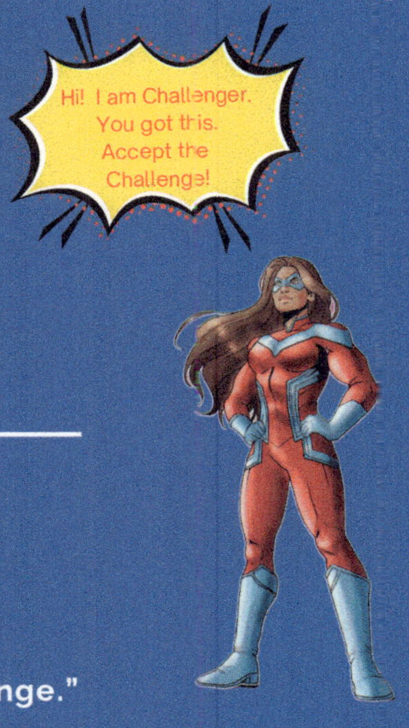

Challenger

____

SIGN HERE

"Every instance of change starts with a challenge."
Accept the Challenge

"EVERY INSTANCE OF CHANGE STARTS WITH A CHALLENGE"

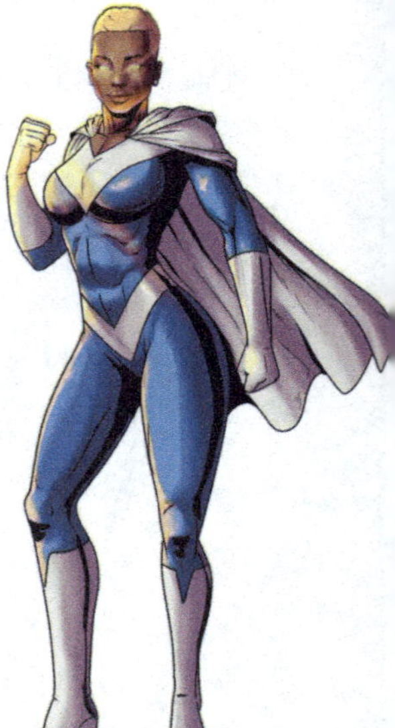

Visionary

How to Use This Journal

Pre-Challenge Work

To get started, identify something that you are currently dealing with that s causing difficulty at home, school, or in your social setting. For the greatest impact, whatever you select must be something that you desire to gradually work on over the next 30 days to achieve the desired change. You will label this as your challenge or goal.

Step 1: Next, think about your PURPOSE for selecting this goal. Consider the following four questions as it relates to the selected challenge or goal:

- Why is addressing this challenge important to you?
- How will addressing this challenge make your life better?
- What do you want to see as a result of addressing this challenge?

Note: If you are unable to answer the questions fully, please consider selecting another challenge to address.

Step 2: Now, reflect on the selected challenge or goal, and identify something(s) about your thinking and behavior that you will need to LET IN (BOUNDARIES) or acknowledge to achieve your desired change. Below are a few thoughts that may be helpful:

- I know that I can do this ....
- I will have to start doing more of....
- I acknowledge I will have to do less of or stop doing ....

How to use this journal (cont):

Step 3: Next, identify something that you will have to EXCUSE YOURSELF (TIME MANAGEMENT) from to achieve the desired change. Below are three questions you must consider.

- What is something I need to stop doing (EXCUSE ME) that may be hindering my progress?
- Who is someone that I need to spend less time with (EXCUSE ME) that may be hindering my progress?

Step 4: Think of some activities or opportunities (ACTIVATORS) you will have to engage in to reach your desired change? Questions to consider:

- What do I need to start doing or spend more time doing that will help my desired change?
- What will it take for me to be successful at doing this new thing(s)?

Step 5: Last, who are the individuals, family, friends, or classmates that can support your (GRAVITATORS) in the journey to desired change? Questions to consider:

- Who is someone I need to spend less time with that may keep me from my desired change?
- Is there someone that I need to stop interacting with (excuse myself from) that may be/will be hindering my progress?

Now, let's practice!

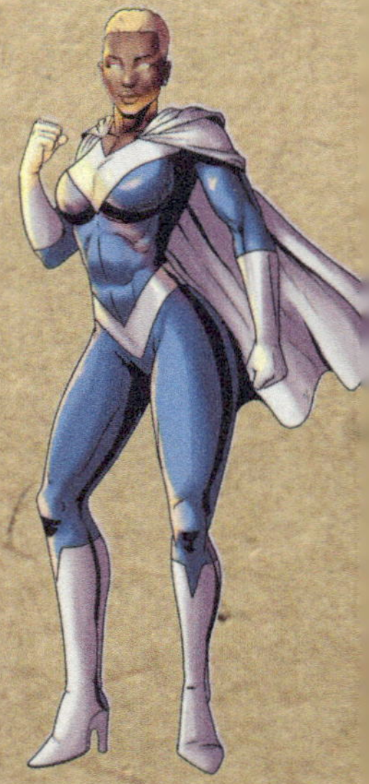

Visionary

ACCEPT THE CHALLENGE
DAILY AFFIRMATION

Today . . .

- I will embrace all challenges (decisions) with a positive mindset.
- I am one challenge away from a change with every challenge I face today.
- I will challenge myself to do something every day that puts me one step closer to my desired change.
- I will build energy from what is fueling my need for change.
- I will only seek opportunities and connect with the individuals that support my change.
- I will be better than I was the day before.
- I celebrate ME because I am enough.
- I accept the challenge.

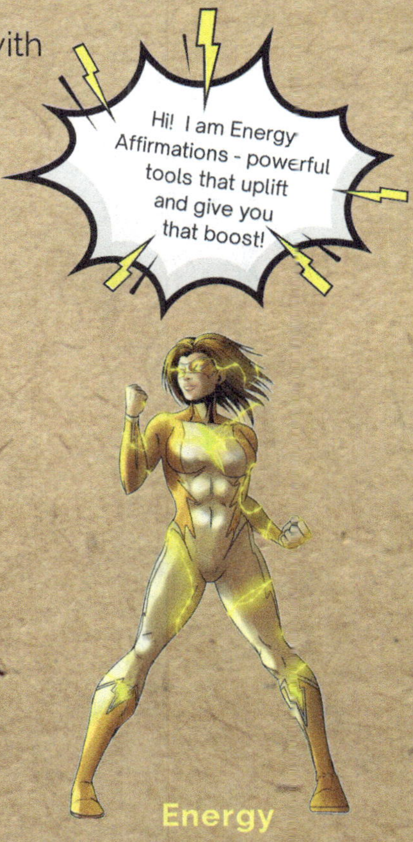

"CHALLENGE OPENS THE DOOR TO CREATE CHANGE.

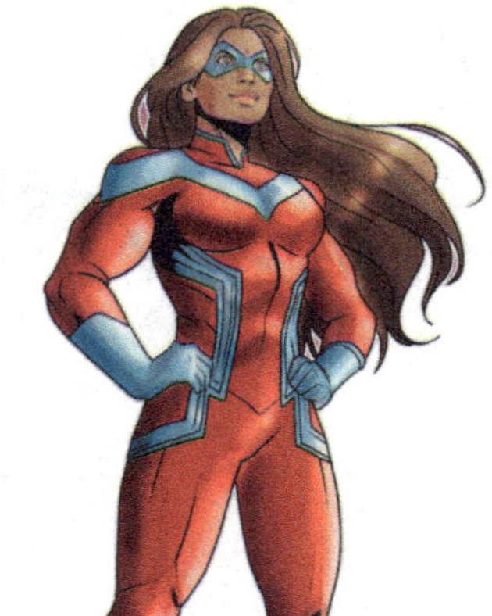

Challenger

THE CHALLENGE

I accept the challenge to:

____

____

LIVE FOR (PURPOSE)

My purpose for addressing this challenge is to:

____

____

LET IN (BOUNDARIES)

To address the challenge, I will let in the following (i.e. activities, people, events).

____

____

EXCUSE ME (TIME MANAGEMENT)

In order to address the challenge, I will not do or do less of the following.

____

____

ACTIVATOR (OPPORTUNITY)

To address the challenge, I will engage in the following activities.

____

____

GRAVITATOR (RELATIONSHIP)

To address the challenge, I will gravitate to the individuals and/or places.

____

____

#EXCUSE ME WHILE I WORK ON ME

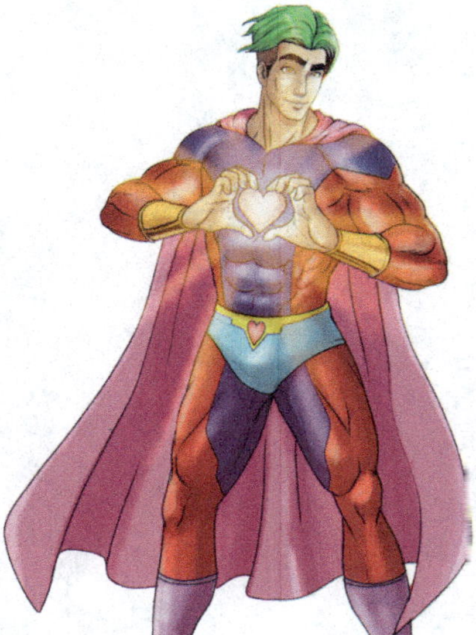

Grateful

Week 1

embrace the
change
today

THE CHALLENGE

I accept the challenge to:

____

LIVE FOR (PURPOSE)

My purpose for reaching my goal is to:

____

LET IN (BOUNDARIES)

In order to reached my goal I will:

____

EXCUSE ME (TIME)

In order to reach my goal, I will:

____

ACTIVATOR (OPPORTUNITY)

In order to reached my goal I will start:

____

GRAVITATOR (RELATIONSHIP)

In order to reached my goal I will connect:

____

When things
change inside,
things change
around you
Sparkle

Date/Time: ______________________

Week 1

Take a moment today to contemplate your challenge (goal), the change you desire (the reason behind it), and the progress you've made. Consider the following aspects:

- What did/do you need to embrace?
- What did/should you excuse yourself from?
- Which opportunities did you/do you need to activate?
- Who did you/do you need to gravitate toward for support?

LIVE FOR (GOAL)

LET IN

EXCUSE ME

ACTIVATE

GRAVITATE

Week 1

Date/Time: ____________________

Take a moment today to contemplate your challenge (goal), the change you desire (the reason behind it), and the progress you've made. Consider the following aspects:

- What did/do you need to embrace?
- What did/should you excuse yourself from?
- Which opportunities did you/do you need to activate?
- Who did you/do you need to gravitate toward for support?

LIVE FOR (GOAL)

LET IN

EXCUSE ME

ACTIVATE

GRAVITATE

Week 1

Date/Time: ____________________

Take a moment today to contemplate your challenge (goal), the change you desire (the reason behind it), and the progress you've made. Consider the following aspects:

- What did/do you need to embrace?
- What did/should you excuse yourself from?
- Which opportunities did you/do you need to activate?
- Who did you/do you need to gravitate toward for support?

LIVE FOR (GOAL)

LET IN

EXCUSE ME

ACTIVATE

GRAVITATE

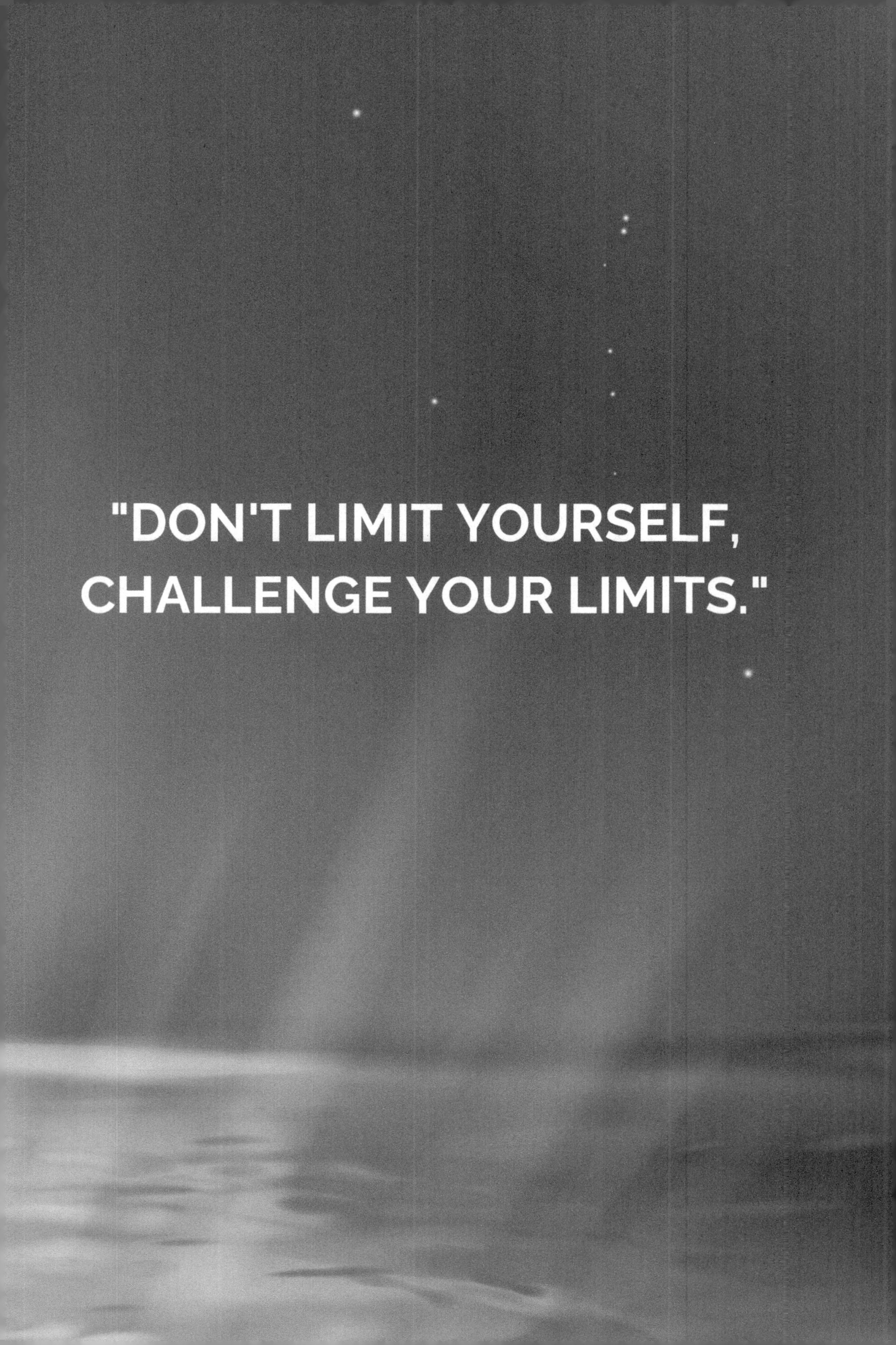
"DON'T LIMIT YOURSELF,
CHALLENGE YOUR LIMITS."

Date/Time: ____________________

Week 1

Take a moment today to contemplate your challenge (goal), the change you desire (the reason behind it), and the progress you've made. Consider the following aspects:

- What did/do you need to embrace?
- What did/should you excuse yourself from?
- Which opportunities did you/do you need to activate?
- Who did you/do you need to gravitate toward for support?

LIVE FOR (GOAL)

LET IN

EXCUSE ME

ACTIVATE

GRAVITATE

Week 1

Date/Time: ______________________

Take a moment today to contemplate your challenge (goal), the change you desire (the reason behind it), and the progress you've made. Consider the following aspects:

- What did/do you need to embrace?
- What did/should you excuse yourself from?
- Which opportunities did you/do you need to activate?
- Who did you/do you need to gravitate toward for support?

LIVE FOR (GOAL)

LET IN

EXCUSE ME

ACTIVATE

GRAVITATE

“ EVERY JOURNEY NEEDS A FIRST STEP

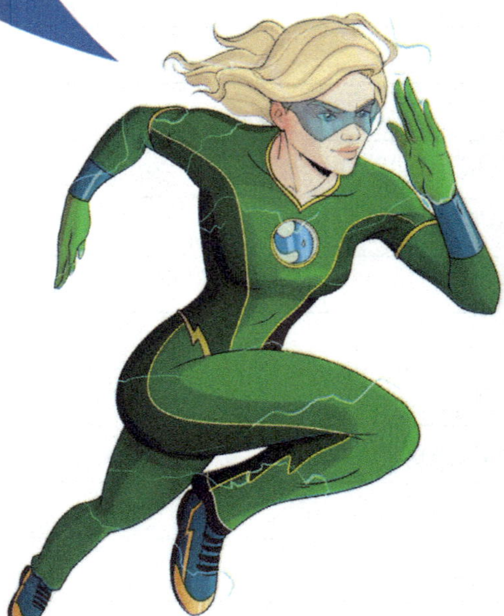

Activator

WEEK 1

CHALLENGE ACCEPTED

GRAVITATOR

of the week

TO:____________________________________

FROM: ____________________________________

KEEP FOR YOUR RECORDS

CHALLENGE ACCEPTED

GRAVITATOR

of the week

TO:____________________________________

FROM: ____________________________________

GIVE TO YOUR GRAVITATOR

CHALLENGE ACCEPTED

EXCUSE ME

for the week

TO:____________________________________

FROM: ____________________________________

GIVE AWAY

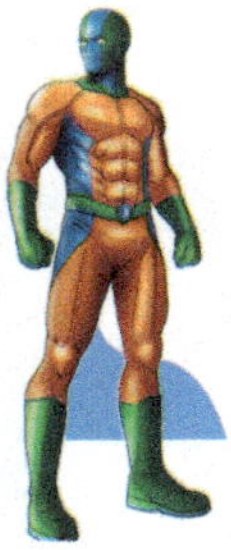

Excusor

REFLECTION
Week 1

Reflect on your week. Share what you are most proud of that put you one step closer to your desired change

OPPORTUNITIES

LET IN (MOST IMPACTFUL)

ACTIVATORS (MOST ENGAGING)

EXCUSE ME (MOST IMPACTFUL

GRAVTATORS (MOST SUPPORTIVE)

Every instance of change starts with a challenge.
Get to the Heart of the challenge.

Week 2

embrace the
change
today

"IF IT DOESN'T CHALLENGE YOU, IT WILL NOT CHANGE YOU"

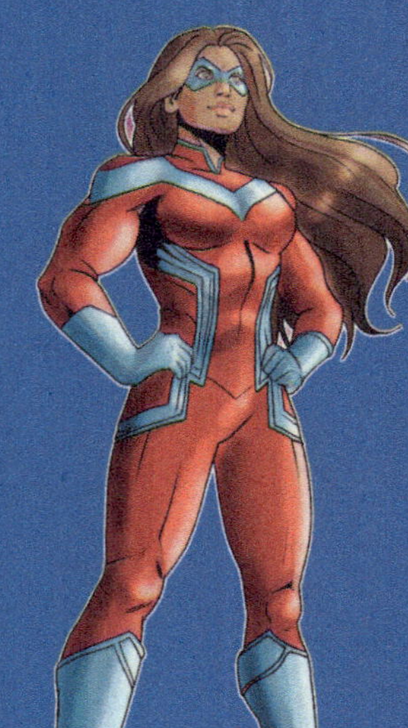

Challenger

THE CHALLENGE

I accept the challenge to:

____

LIVE FOR (PURPOSE)

My purpose for reaching my goal is to:

____

LET IN (BOUNDARIES)

In order to reached my goal I will:

____

EXCUSE ME (TIME)

In order to reach my goal, I will:

____

ACTIVATOR (OPPORTUNITY)

In order to reached my goal I will start:

____

GRAVITATOR (RELATIONSHIP)

In order to reached my goal I will connect:

____

Week 2

Date/Time: ____________________

Take a moment today to contemplate your challenge (goal), the change you desire (the reason behind it), and the progress you've made. Consider the following aspects:

- What did/do you need to embrace?
- What did/should you excuse yourself from?
- Which opportunities did you/do you need to activate?
- Who did you/do you need to gravitate toward for support?

LIVE FOR (GOAL)

LET IN

EXCUSE ME

ACTIVATE

GRAVITATE

Date/Time: ____________________

Week 2

Take a moment today to contemplate your challenge (goal), the change you desire (the reason behind it), and the progress you've made. Consider the following aspects:

- What did/do you need to embrace?
- What did/should you excuse yourself from?
- Which opportunities did you/do you need to activate?
- Who did you/do you need to gravitate toward for support?

LIVE FOR (GOAL)

LET IN

EXCUSE ME

ACTIVATE

GRAVITATE

Date/Time: ______________________

Week 2

Take a moment today to contemplate your challenge (goal), the change you desire (the reason behind it), and the progress you've made. Consider the following aspects:

- What did/do you need to embrace?
- What did/should you excuse yourself from?
- Which opportunities did you/do you need to activate?
- Who did you/do you need to gravitate toward for support?

LIVE FOR (GOAL)

LET IN

EXCUSE ME

ACTIVATE

GRAVITATE

keep
activating those
opportunities

Week 2

Date/Time: ____________________

Take a moment today to contemplate your challenge (goal), the change you desire (the reason behind it), and the progress you've made. Consider the following aspects:

- What did/do you need to embrace?
- What did/should you excuse yourself from?
- Which opportunities did you/do you need to activate?
- Who did you/do you need to gravitate toward for support?

LIVE FOR (GOAL)

LET IN

EXCUSE ME

ACTIVATE

GRAVITATE

Date/Time: ______________________

Week 2

Take a moment today to contemplate your challenge (goal), the change you desire (the reason behind it), and the progress you've made. Consider the following aspects:

- What did/do you need to embrace?
- What did/should you excuse yourself from?
- Which opportunities did you/do you need to activate?
- Who did you/do you need to gravitate toward for support?

LIVE FOR (GOAL)

LET IN

EXCUSE ME

ACTIVATE

GRAVITATE

WOO-HOO!
Half way there.

WEEK 2

CHALLENGE ACCEPTED

GRAVITATOR

of the week

TO:______________________________

FROM: ___________________________

KEEP FOR YOUR RECORDS

CHALLENGE ACCEPTED

GRAVITATOR

of the week

TO:______________________________

FROM: ___________________________

GIVE TO YOUR GRAVITATOR

CHALLENGE ACCEPTED

EXCUSE ME

for the week

TO:______________________________

FROM: ___________________________

GIVE AWAY

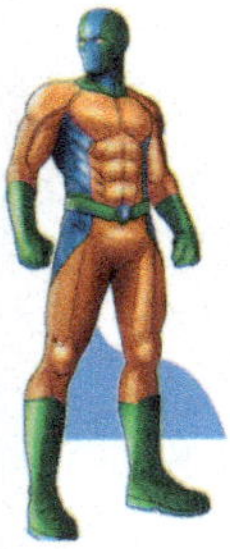

Excusor

REFLECTION
Week 2

Reflect on your week. Share what you are most proud of that put you one step closer to your desired change

OPPORTUNITIES

LET IN (MOST IMPACTFUL)

ACTIVATORS (MOST ENGAGING)

EXCUSE ME (MOST IMPACTFUL

GRAVTATORS (MOST SUPPORTIVE)

Every instance of change starts with a challenge.
Get to the Heart of the challenge.

Week 3

embrace the *change* today

THE CHALLENGE

I accept the challenge to:

____

LIVE FOR (PURPOSE)

My purpose for reaching my goal is to:

____

LET IN (BOUNDARIES)

In order to reached my goal I will:

____

EXCUSE ME (TIME)

In order to reach my goal, I will:

____

ACTIVATOR (OPPORTUNITY)

In order to reached my goal I will start:

____

GRAVITATOR (RELATIONSHIP)

In order to reached my goal I will connect:

____

Date/Time: ______________________

Week 3

Take a moment today to contemplate your challenge (goal), the change you desire (the reason behind it), and the progress you've made. Consider the following aspects:

- What did/do you need to embrace?
- What did/should you excuse yourself from?
- Which opportunities did you/do you need to activate?
- Who did you/do you need to gravitate toward for support?

LIVE FOR (GOAL)

LET IN

EXCUSE ME

ACTIVATE

GRAVITATE

Week 3

Date/Time: ____________________

Take a moment today to contemplate your challenge (goal), the change you desire (the reason behind it), and the progress you've made. Consider the following aspects:

- What did/do you need to embrace?
- What did/should you excuse yourself from?
- Which opportunities did you/do you need to activate?
- Who did you/do you need to gravitate toward for support?

LIVE FOR (GOAL)

LET IN

EXCUSE ME

ACTIVATE

GRAVITATE

Week 3

Date/Time: ______________________

Take a moment today to contemplate your challenge (goal), the change you desire (the reason behind it), and the progress you've made. Consider the following aspects:

- What did/do you need to embrace?
- What did/should you excuse yourself from?
- Which opportunities did you/do you need to activate?
- Who did you/do you need to gravitate toward for support?

LIVE FOR (GOAL)

LET IN

EXCUSE ME

ACTIVATE

GRAVITATE

you are a *limited* edition
change starts with you.

Date/Time: ______________________

Week 3

Take a moment today to contemplate your challenge (goal), the change you desire (the reason behind it), and the progress you've made. Consider the following aspects:

- What did/do you need to embrace?
- What did/should you excuse yourself from?
- Which opportunities did you/do you need to activate?
- Who did you/do you need to gravitate toward for support?

LIVE FOR (GOAL)

LET IN

EXCUSE ME

ACTIVATE

GRAVITATE

Week 3

Date/Time: ____________________

Take a moment today to contemplate your challenge (goal), the change you desire (the reason behind it), and the progress you've made. Consider the following aspects:

- What did/do you need to embrace?
- What did/should you excuse yourself from?
- Which opportunities did you/do you need to activate?
- Who did you/do you need to gravitate toward for support?

LIVE FOR (GOAL)

LET IN

EXCUSE ME

ACTIVATE

GRAVITATE

"IT TAKES TIME TO ACHIEVE GREATNESS."

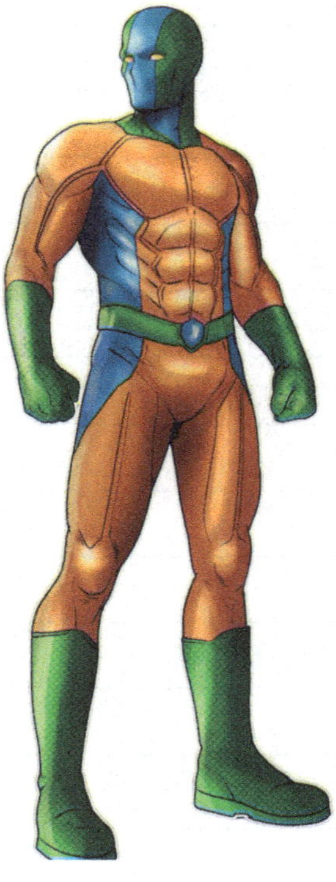

Excusor

change begins at
the end of your comfort zone

Roy T. Bennett

WEEK 3

CHALLENGE ACCEPTED

GRAVITATOR
of the week

TO:______________________________

FROM: ____________________________

KEEP FOR YOUR RECORDS

CHALLENGE ACCEPTED

GRAVITATOR
of the week

TO:______________________________

FROM: ____________________________

GIVE TO YOUR GRAVITATOR

CHALLENGE ACCEPTED

EXCUSE ME
for the week

TO:______________________________

FROM: ____________________________

GIVE AWAY

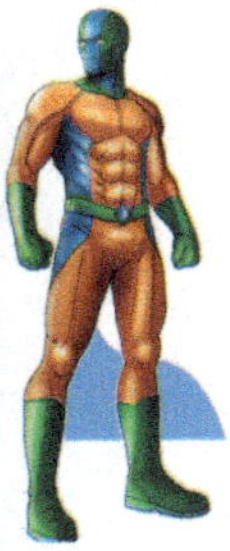

Excusor

REFLECTION
Week 3

Reflect on your week. Share what you are most proud of that put you one step closer to your desired change

OPPORTUNITIES

LET IN (MOST IMPACTFUL)

ACTIVATORS (MOST ENGAGING)

EXCUSE ME (MOST IMPACTFUL

GRAVTATORS (MOST SUPPORTIVE)

Every instance of change starts with a challenge.
Get to the Heart of the challenge.

Week 4

embrace the
change
today

THE CHALLENGE

I accept the challenge to:

____

LIVE FOR (PURPOSE)

My purpose for reaching my goal is to:

____

LET IN (BOUNDARIES)

In order to reached my goal I will:

____

EXCUSE ME (TIME)

In order to reach my goal, I will:

___

ACTIVATOR (OPPORTUNITY)

In order to reached my goal I will start:

___

GRAVITATOR (RELATIONSHIP)

In order to reached my goal I will connect:

___

Date/Time: ____________________

Week 4

Take a moment today to contemplate your challenge (goal), the change you desire (the reason behind it), and the progress you've made. Consider the following aspects:

- What did/do you need to embrace?
- What did/should you excuse yourself from?
- Which opportunities did you/do you need to activate?
- Who did you/do you need to gravitate toward for support?

LIVE FOR (GOAL)

LET IN

EXCUSE ME

ACTIVATE

GRAVITATE

Week 4

Date/Time: ____________________

Take a moment today to contemplate your challenge (goal), the change you desire (the reason behind it), and the progress you've made. Consider the following aspects:

- What did/do you need to embrace?
- What did/should you excuse yourself from?
- Which opportunities did you/do you need to activate?
- Who did you/do you need to gravitate toward for support?

LIVE FOR (GOAL)

LET IN

EXCUSE ME

ACTIVATE

GRAVITATE

Week 4

Date/Time: ____________________

Take a moment today to contemplate your challenge (goal), the change you desire (the reason behind it), and the progress you've made. Consider the following aspects:

- What did/do you need to embrace?
- What did/should you excuse yourself from?
- Which opportunities did you/do you need to activate?
- Who did you/do you need to gravitate toward for support?

LIVE FOR (GOAL)

LET IN

EXCUSE ME

ACTIVATE

GRAVITATE

keep
looking for
activators

Date/Time: ______________________

Week 4

Take a moment today to contemplate your challenge (goal), the change you desire (the reason behind it), and the progress you've made. Consider the following aspects:

- What did/do you need to embrace?
- What did/should you excuse yourself from?
- Which opportunities did you/do you need to activate?
- Who did you/do you need to gravitate toward for support?

LIVE FOR (GOAL)

LET IN

EXCUSE ME

ACTIVATE

GRAVITATE

Date/Time: ____________________

Week 4

Take a moment today to contemplate your challenge (goal), the change you desire (the reason behind it), and the progress you've made. Consider the following aspects:

- What did/do you need to embrace?
- What did/should you excuse yourself from?
- Which opportunities did you/do you need to activate?
- Who did you/do you need to gravitate toward for support?

LIVE FOR (GOAL)

LET IN

EXCUSE ME

ACTIVATE

GRAVITATE

change loading....

“

KEEP PUSHING

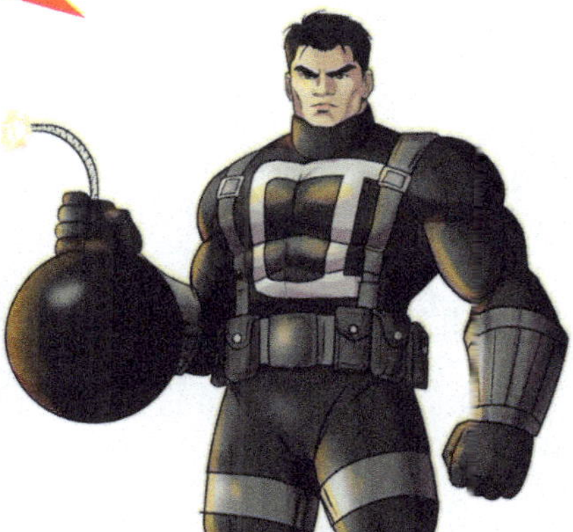

Detonator

WEEK 4

CHALLENGE ACCEPTED

GRAVITATOR
of the week

TO:______________________________

FROM: ____________________________

KEEP FOR YOUR RECORDS

CHALLENGE ACCEPTED

GRAVITATOR
of the week

TO:______________________________

FROM: ____________________________

GIVE TO YOUR GRAVITATOR

CHALLENGE ACCEPTED

EXCUSE ME
for the week

TO:______________________________

FROM: ____________________________

GIVE AWAY

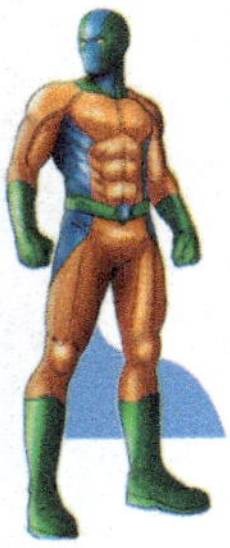

Excusor

REFLECTION
Week 4

Reflect on your week. Share what you are most proud of that put you one step closer to your desired change

OPPORTUNITIES

LET IN (MOST IMPACTFUL)

ACTIVATORS (MOST ENGAGING)

EXCUSE ME (MOST IMPACTFUL

GRAVTATORS (MOST SUPPORTIVE)

Every instance of change starts with a challenge.
Get to the Heart of the challenge.

Week 5

embrace the
change
today

THE CHALLENGE

I accept the challenge to:

____

LIVE FOR (PURPOSE)

My purpose for reaching my goal is to:

____

LET IN (BOUNDARIES)

In order to reached my goal I will:

____

EXCUSE ME (TIME)

In order to reach my goal, I will:

____

ACTIVATOR (OPPORTUNITY)

In order to reached my goal I will start:

____

GRAVITATOR (RELATIONSHIP)

In order to reached my goal I will connect:

____

Date/Time: ____________________

Week 5

Take a moment today to contemplate your challenge (goal), the change yo desire (the reason behind it), and the progress you've made. Consider the following aspects:

- What did/do you need to embrace?
- What did/should you excuse yourself from?
- Which opportunities did you/do you need to activate?
- Who did you/do you need to gravitate toward for support?

LIVE FOR (GOAL)

LET IN

EXCUSE ME

ACTIVATE

GRAVITATE

Week 5

Date/Time: ______________________

Take a moment today to contemplate your challenge (goal), the change you desire (the reason behind it), and the progress you've made. Consider the following aspects:

- What did/do you need to embrace?
- What did/should you excuse yourself from?
- Which opportunities did you/do you need to activate?
- Who did you/do you need to gravitate toward for support?

LIVE FOR (GOAL)

LET IN

EXCUSE ME

ACTIVATE

GRAVITATE

Date/Time: ______________________

Week 5

Take a moment today to contemplate your challenge (goal), the change you desire (the reason behind it), and the progress you've made. Consider the following aspects:

- What did/do you need to embrace?
- What did/should you excuse yourself from?
- Which opportunities did you/do you need to activate?
- Who did you/do you need to gravitate toward for support?

LIVE FOR (GOAL)

LET IN

EXCUSE ME

ACTIVATE

GRAVITATE

positive steps,
make positive change

Week 5

Date/Time: ______________________

Take a moment today to contemplate your challenge (goal), the change yo desire (the reason behind it), and the progress you've made. Consider the following aspects:

- What did/do you need to embrace?
- What did/should you excuse yourself from?
- Which opportunities did you/do you need to activate?
- Who did you/do you need to gravitate toward for support?

LIVE FOR (GOAL)

LET IN

EXCUSE ME

ACTIVATE

GRAVITATE

Week 5

Date/Time: ____________________

Take a moment today to contemplate your challenge (goal), the change you desire (the reason behind it), and the progress you've made. Consider the following aspects:

- What did/do you need to embrace?
- What did/should you excuse yourself from?
- Which opportunities did you/do you need to activate?
- Who did you/do you need to gravitate toward for support?

LIVE FOR (GOAL)

LET IN

EXCUSE ME

ACTIVATE

GRAVITATE

Use this moment to celebrate your change!

"You have to change
your thinking
if you desire to have a
future different
from your present."

— Germany Kent

WEEK 5

CHALLENGE ACCEPTED

GRAVITATOR
of the week

TO:_______________________________

FROM: ____________________________

KEEP FOR YOUR RECORDS

CHALLENGE ACCEPTED

GRAVITATOR
of the week

TO:_______________________________

FROM: ____________________________

GIVE TO YOUR GRAVITATOR

CHALLENGE ACCEPTED

EXCUSE ME
for the week

TO:_______________________________

FROM: ____________________________

GIVE AWAY

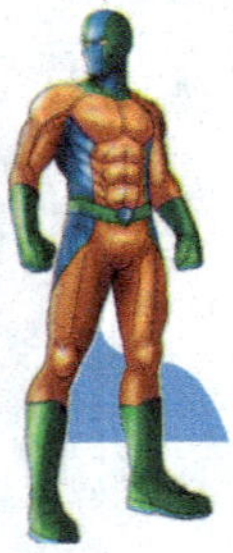

Excusor

REFLECTION
Week 5

Reflect on your week. Share what you are most proud of that put you one step closer to your desired change

OPPORTUNITIES

LET IN (MOST IMPACTFUL)

ACTIVATORS (MOST ENGAGING)

EXCUSE ME (MOST IMPACTFUL

GRAVTATORS (MOST SUPPORTIVE)

Every instance of change starts with a challenge.
Get to the Heart of the challenge.

ACTIVATOR TRACKER

Log your daily opportunities/activities that you engaged in or excused yourself from to support your efforts to reach your goal.

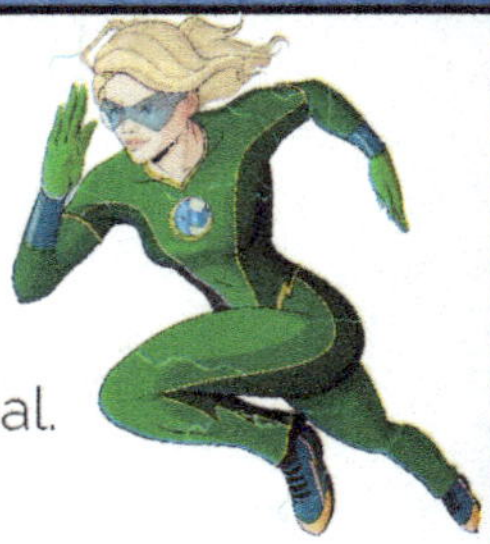

Activator

DATE	OPPORTUNITY/ACTIVITY	HOW DID YOU FEEL? HAPPY? SAD?

Get the supplies you need now to build reslience and grow in life.

#activators
#gravitators

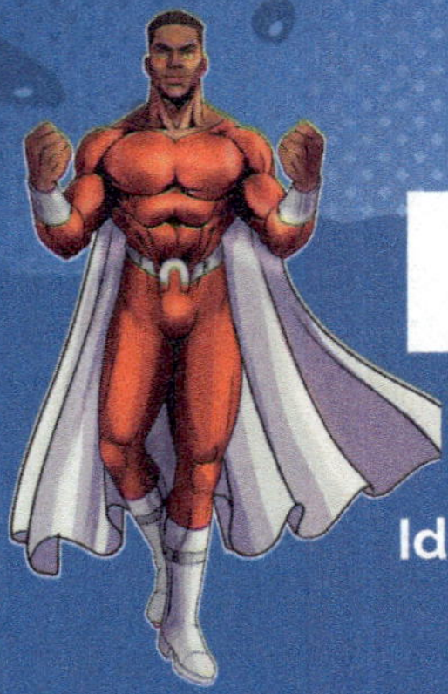

Gravitator

GRAVITATOR TRACKER

Identify at least one person that supported you today in addressing the challenge.

Gravitator Name	Relationship	Phone	✓
			☐
			☐
			☐
			☐
			☐
			☐
			☐
			☐
			☐
			☐
			☐
			☐
			☐

"Once your mindset changes, everything on the outside will change along with it."

~ Steve Maraboli

FREE WRITE

FREE WRITE

almost there, don't give up

FREE WRITI

permit the

change...

FREE WRITE

Who have you gravitated to?

FREE WRITI

"You have to change
your thinking
if you desire to have a
future different
from your present."

— Germany Kent

FREE WRITE

currently making

change...

FREE WRIT

positive steps,
make positive change

FREE WRITE

"CHANGE RESULTS IN PROGRESSION FORWARD.

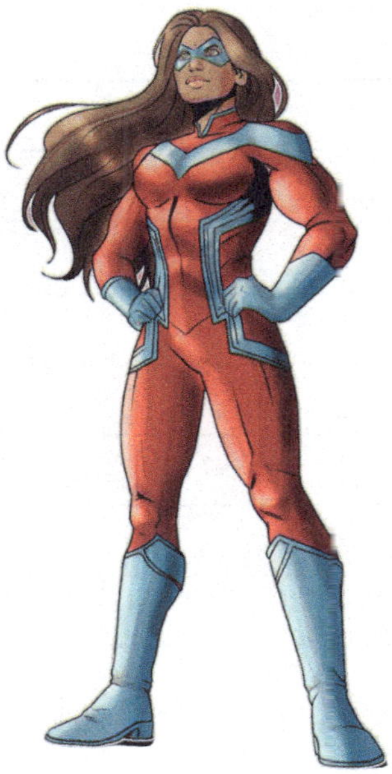

Challenger

FREE WRITI

locking in the *change...*

FREE WRITE

Have you considered who you could be a gravitator for?

close never feels close
until you're nearly there

FREE WRITE

“

CHANGE IS LIKE A PENNY; KEEP IT AND IT ADDS UP OVER TIME.

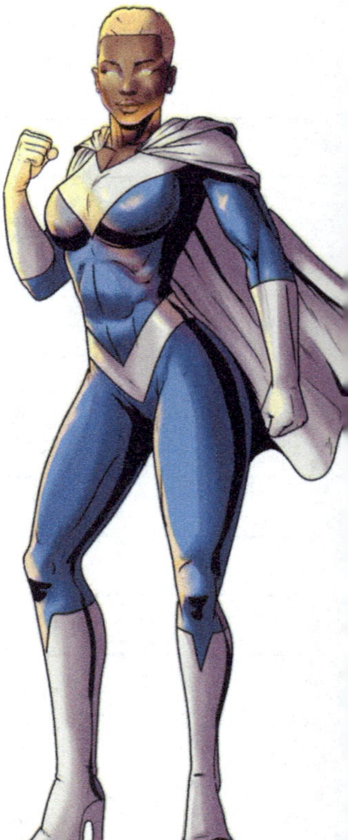

Visionary

FREE WRITE

change...
made

FREE WRITE

Thank you notes are a quick way to show a gravitator that you appreciate them.

FREE WRITE

FREE WRITI

FREE WRITE

FREE WRITE

FREE WRITE

FREE WRITI

FREE WRITE

FREE WRITE

FREE WRITE

FREE WRITI

FREE WRITE

FREE WRITE

FREE WRITE

FREE WRIT

FREE WRITE

FREE WRITE

FREE WRITE

FREE WRITI

FREE WRITE

FREE WRITE

FREE WRITE

FREE WRIT

FREE WRITE

FREE WRITE

FREE WRITE

welcome to

your New You

WAY TO GO!

You just completed the

ACCEPT THE CHALLENGE Workbook

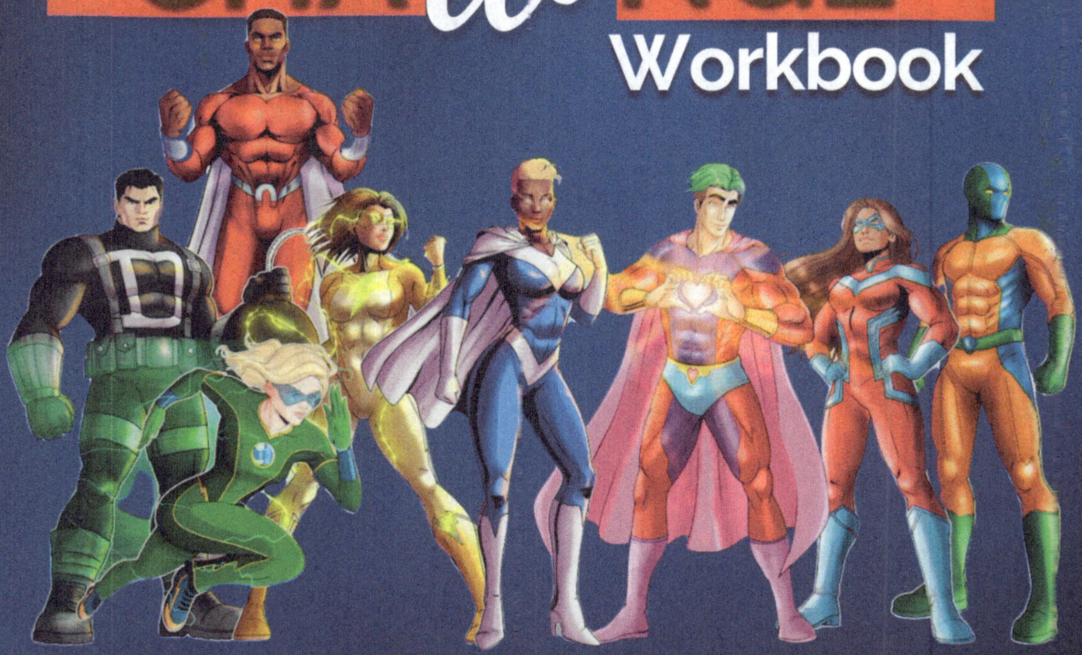

Now, you're ready for more!
Let's level it up a notch...
You're ready to say:

CHALLENGE ACCEPTED

Every instance of change starts with a challenge.
Get to the Heart of the challenge.

"The greatest discovery of all time is that a person can change his future by merely changing his attitude."

-OPRAH WINFREY

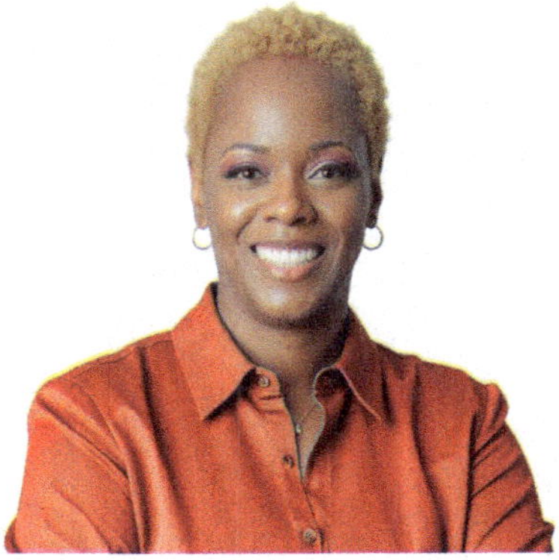

About Us

The Gordon Visionary Journals Series offers a distinct and thought-provoking approach to journaling through unique prompts. By incorporating the Gordon Visionary Journals into your routine, you are adding a valuable tool to help you achieve your goals and lead a purposeful life.

Trisha R. Gordon, founder and visionary behind Gordon Visionary Journals, she a devoted believer, published author, inspirational speaker, mentor, and philanthropist, inspires individuals with her uplifting messages, writing, and journal collection. Her innovative perspective on redefining words to transform life illustrates how adversity can be a stepping stone to success by approaching life's challenges with a positive mindset.

RedefinHER

Made in the USA
Coppell, TX
21 June 2026

82781212R10085